Arthritis

All That You Need To Know About The Anti-Inflamatory Diet For Treating Arthritis Pain Relief, Groin Pain, Bursitis, Knee Pain, PFS, AKPS.

Cherilyn K. Chaffin

Table of Contents

ARTHRITIS 1

INTRODUCTION 4

CHAPTER 1 5

    ARTHRITIS 5
    FAST FACTS ON ARTHRITIS 6
    TREATMENT 7

CHAPTER 2 9

    MEDICATION 9
        Natural Remedies 11
        Foods to avoid 12
        Physical therapies 15
        Physical activity 16
        Natural Therapies 17
        Causes of arthritis 18
        Risk factors for arthritis 20

CHAPTER 3 57

    9 HERBS TO BATTLE ARTHRITIS PAIN 57
    ASK YOUR PHYSICIAN ABOUT COMPLEMENTARY MEDICINE 63

ACKNOWLEDGEMENTS 66

Copyright © 2022 by Cherilyn K. Chaffin

All rights reserved. No part of this publication may be reproduced, distributed, or transmitted in any form or by any means, including photocopying, recording, or other electronic or mechanical methods, without the prior written permission of the publisher, except in the case of brief quotations embodied in critical reviews and certain other non-commercial uses permitted by copyright law.

Introduction

Joint disease is the inflammation and tenderness of one or more of your bones. The primary symptoms of joint disease are joint pain and tightness, which typically get worse with age. The most frequent types of joint disease are osteoarthritis and arthritis rheumatoid.

Osteoarthritis causes cartilage - the hard, slippery cells that addresses the ends of bone fragments where they form a joint - to breakdown. Arthritis rheumatoid is an illness where the immune system episodes the joints, you start with the liner of joints.

The crystals, which form when there's too much the crystals in your blood, can cause gout. Infections or root disease, such as psoriasis or lupus, can cause other styles of arthritis.

Treatments vary with respect to the type of joint disease. The primary goals of joint disease treatments are to lessen symptoms and improve standard of living.

Chapter 1

Arthritis

Joint disease is the inflammation and tenderness of one or more of your bones. The primary symptoms of joint disease are joint pain and tightness, which typically get worse with age. The most frequent types of joint disease are osteoarthritis and arthritis rheumatoid.

Osteoarthritis causes cartilage - the hard, slippery cells that addresses the ends of bone fragments where they form a joint - to breakdown. Arthritis rheumatoid is an illness where the immune system episodes the joints, you start with the liner of joints.

The crystals, which form when there's too much the crystals in your blood, can cause gout. Infections or root disease, such as psoriasis or lupus, can cause other styles of arthritis.

Treatments vary with respect to the type of joint disease.

The primary goals of joint disease treatments are to lessen symptoms and improve standard of living.

Fast facts on arthritis

Below are a few tips about arthritis. Greater detail is within the primary article.

- Arthritis identifies around 200 rheumatic diseases and conditions that impact joint parts, including lupus and arthritis rheumatoid.

- It can result in a selection of symptoms and impair someone's ability to execute everyday tasks.

- Exercise has an optimistic influence on arthritis and can improve pain, function, and mental health.

- Factors in the introduction of arthritis include damage, abnormal metabolism, genetic make-up, infections, and disease fighting capability dysfunction.

- Treatment aims to regulate pain, minimize joint

harm, and improve or maintain standard of living. It entails medications, physical therapies, and patient education and support.

Treatment

Treatment for joint disease aims to regulate pain, minimize joint harm, and improve or maintain function and standard of living.

A variety of medications and lifestyle strategies can help accomplish that and protect important joints from further harm.

Treatment might involve:

- medications
- non-pharmacologic therapies
- physical or occupational therapy
- splints or joint assistive aids
- patient education and support

- weight loss

- surgery, including joint replacement

Chapter 2

Medication

noninflammatory types of arthritis, such as osteoarthritis, tend to be treated with pain-reducing medications, exercise, weight reduction if the individual is obese, and self-management education.

These treatments are also put on inflammatory types of arthritis, such as RA, along with anti-inflammatory medications such as corticosteroids and nonsteroidal anti-inflammatory drugs (NSAIDs), disease-modifying anti-rheumatic drugs (DMARDs), and a comparatively new class of drugs known as biologics.

Medications depends on the kind of arthritis. Popular drugs include:

- Analgesics: these decrease pain, but haven't any effect on swelling. For example acetaminophen (Tylenol), tramadol (Ultram) and narcotics that contains oxycodone (Percocet, Oxycontin) or hydrocodone (Vicodin, Lortab). Tylenol is available to buy online.

- nonsteroidal anti-inflammatory drugs (NSAIDs): these reduce both pain and inflammation. NSAIDs include available to buy over-the-counter or online, includeing ibuprofen (Advil, Motrin IB) and naproxen sodium (Aleve). Some NSAIDs can be found as lotions, gels or areas which may be put on specific joints.

- Counterirritants: some ointments and creams contain menthol or capsaicin, the component that makes chile peppers spicy. Massaging these on your skin over an agonizing joint can modulate pain indicators from the joint and reduce pain. Various lotions are available to buy online.

- Disease-modifying antirheumatic drugs (DMARDs): used to take care of RA, DMARDs sluggish or stop the disease fighting capability from attacking the bones. For example methotrexate (Trexall) and hydroxychloroquine (Plaquenil).

- Biologics: used in combination with DMARDs, biologic response modifiers are genetically engineered drugs that focus on various protein substances mixed up in immune response. For example etanercept (Enbrel) and infliximab (Remicade).

- Corticosteroids: prednisone and cortisone reduce irritation and suppress the disease fighting capability.

Natural Remedies

A healthful, balanced diet with appropriate exercise, avoiding smoking, rather than taking in excess alcohol can help people who have arthritis maintain their general health.

Diet

There is absolutely no specific diet that treats arthritis,

however, many types of food can help reduce inflammation.

The next foods, within a Mediterranean diet, can offer many nutrients that are best for joint health:

- Fish.
- nut products and seeds.
- fruits & vegetables.
- Beans.
- olive oil.
- whole grains

Foods to avoid

There are a few foods that individuals with arthritis may choose to avoid.

Nightshade vegetables, such as tomato vegetables, contain a chemical substance called solanine that some studies have associated with joint disease pain. Research results are mixed as it pertains to these vegetables, but many people have reported a decrease in joint disease symptoms when staying away from nightshade vegetables.

Self-management

Self-management of joint disease symptoms is also important.

Key strategies include:

- remaining physically active.
- achieving and keeping a wholesome weight.
- getting regular check-ups with the physician.
- protecting bones from unnecessary stress

Seven habits that will help a person with arthritis to control their condition are:

1. Organization: keep an eye on symptoms, pain quantity, medications, and possible part results for

consultations with your physician..

2. Managing pain and exhaustion: a medication regimen can be coupled with nonmedical pain management. Understanding how to manage exhaustion is paramount to living easily with arthritis..

3. Remaining active: exercise is effective for controlling arthritis and general health.

4. Balancing activity with relax: in addition to staying active, relax is equally important whenever your disease is dynamic.

5. Eating a healthful diet: a well balanced diet will help you achieve a wholesome weight and control inflammation. Avoid processed, processed food items and pro-inflammatory animal-derived foods and choose entire herb foods that are saturated in antioxidants and which have anti-inflammatory properties.

6. Improving rest: poor rest can aggravate arthritis

pain and fatigue. Do something to improve rest hygiene and that means you find it simpler to drift off and stay asleep. Avoid caffeine and intense exercise in the evenings and restrict screen-time right before sleeping.

7. Caring for joint parts: methods for safeguarding bones include using the stronger, larger joint parts as levers when starting doorways, using several bones to spread the weight of the object such as using a back pack and gripping as loosely as you possibly can by using padded deals with.

Do not sit down in the same position for very long periods. Take regular breaks to keep mobile.

Physical therapies

Doctors will most likely recommend a span of physical therapy to help patients with joint disease overcome a few of the difficulties and also to reduce restrictions on mobility.

Types of physical therapy which may be recommended include:

- warm water therapy: exercises in a warm-water pool. Water helps weight and places less strain on the muscles and joints.

- Physical therapy: specific exercises personalized to the problem and specific needs, sometimes coupled with pain-relieving treatments such as ice or hot packs and massage.

- Occupational therapy: useful advice on managing everyday tasks, choosing specific aids and equipment, defending the important joints from further damage and managing fatigue

Physical activity

Research shows that although people with joint disease may experience short-term raises in pain when first starting exercise, continued exercise can be a highly effective way to lessen symptomsTrusted Source long-term.

People with joint disease can take part in joint-friendly exercise independently or with friends. As many folks with joint disease have another condition, such as cardiovascular disease, it's important to choose appropriate activities.

Joint-friendly activities that work for adults with arthritis and cardiovascular disease include:

- Walking.
- Swimming.
- cycling

A healthcare professional can support you in finding ways to live a healthful lifestyle and also have a better standard of living.

Natural Therapies

Several natural treatments have been suggested for different kinds of arthritis.

Based on the organization Versus Arthritis, located in the uk (U.K.), some research has backed the utilization of devil's claw, rosehip, and Boswellia, from the frankincense tree. Devil's claw and Boswellia vitamins can be bought online.

There is certainly some evidenceTrusted Source that turmeric can help, but more studies are had a need to confirm their effectiveness.

Several other herbs and spices have been recommended for RA, but again, more research is necessary. They include turmeric, garlic clove, ginger, dark pepper, and green tea extract.

Several natural herbs and spices can be found to buy online in product form, including turmeric, ginger, and garlic clove.

Anyone who's considering using natural treatments for any kind of joint disease should talk with a health care provider first.

Causes of arthritis

There is absolutely no single reason behind all sorts of arthritis. The reason or causes differ based on the type or form of joint disease.

Possible causes can include:

- injury, resulting in degenerative arthritis.
- abnormal metabolism, resulting in gout and pseudogout.
- inheritance, such as with osteoarthritis.
- infections, such as the joint disease of Lyme disease.
- disease fighting capability dysfunction, such as with RA and SLE

Most types of joint disease are associated with a mixture of factors, however, many have no apparent cause and appearance to be unstable in their introduction.

Some individuals may be genetically much more likely to

build up certain arthritic conditions. Additional factors, such as earlier injury, contamination, smoking and challenging occupations, can connect to genes to help expand increase the threat of arthritis.

Diet and nutrition can are likely involved in managing joint disease and the chance of joint disease, although particular foods, food sensitivities or intolerances aren't recognized to cause arthritis.

Foods that increase swelling, particularly animal-derived foods and diets saturated in refined sugars, can make symptoms even worse, as can eating foodstuffs that provoke an disease fighting capability response.

Gout is one kind of joint disease that is closely associated with diet, as it is caused by elevated degrees of uric acidity which may be due to a diet saturated in purines.

Diets which contain high-purine foods, such as sea food, burgandy or merlot wine, and meat, can result in a gout flare-up. Vegetables and other flower foods which contain high degrees of purines do not may actually exacerbate gout symptoms, however.

Risk factors for arthritis

Certain risk factors have been associated with arthritis. A few of these are modifiable while some are not.

Non-modifiable arthritis risk factors:

- Age: the chance of developing most types of joint disease increases with age group.

- Sex: most types of joint disease are more prevalent in females, and 60 percent of most people with joint disease are woman. Gout is more prevalent in men than females.

- Hereditary factors: specific genes are associated with an increased threat of certain types of arthritis, such as arthritis rheumatoid (RA), systemic lupus erythematosus (SLE) and ankylosing spondylitis.

Modifiable arthritis risk factors:

- Overweight and weight problems: unwanted

weight can donate to both the starting point and development of leg osteoarthritis.

- Joint injuries: harm to a joint can donate to the introduction of osteoarthritis for the reason that joint.

- Contamination: many microbial brokers can infect joint parts and cause the development of varied forms of joint disease.

Profession: certain occupations that involve repetitive leg twisting and squatting are associated with osteoarthritis of the leg.

Comorbidities

Over fifty percent of adults in the U.S. with joint disease report high blood circulation pressure. High blood circulation pressure is associated with cardiovascular disease, the most typical comorbidity among adults with joint disease.

Around 1 in 5 of adults in the U.S. who've joint disease are smokers. Smoking is associated with chronic respiratory conditions, the next most common comorbidity among adults with joint disease.

Types of arthritis

There remain 200 types of arthritis, or musculoskeletal conditions. They are put into seven main organizations:

- Inflammatory arthritis.
- Degenerative or mechanised arthritis.
- Smooth tissue musculoskeletal pain.
- Back pain.
- Connective tissue disease.
- Infectious arthritis.
- Metabolic arthritis.

1. Inflammatory arthritis

Inflammation is a standard area of the body's healing up process. The inflammation will happen as a protection against infections and bacterias or as a reply to accidental injuries such as burns up. However, with inflammatory joint disease, irritation occurs in people for no obvious reason.

Inflammatory joint disease is seen as a damaging inflammation that will not occur as a standard reaction to damage or infection. This sort of swelling is unhelpful and instead causes harm in the affected bones, leading to pain, rigidity and swelling.

Inflammatory arthritis make a difference several bones, and the swelling can damage the top of joints as well as the underlying bone.

Types of inflammatory joint disease include:

- Arthritis rheumatoid (RA)

- Reactive arthritis.

- Ankylosing spondylitis.

- Joint disease associated with colitis or psoriasis

The term "arthritis" means "joint inflammation," but inflammation could also affect the tendons and ligaments surrounding the joint.

2. Degenerative or mechanised arthritis

Degenerative or mechanised arthritis identifies several conditions that mainly involve harm to the cartilage that addresses the ends of the bone fragments.

The primary job of the smooth, slippery cartilage is to help the joints glide and move smoothly. This sort of joint disease causes the cartilage to be slimmer and rougher.

To pay for the increased loss of cartilage and changes in joint function, your body starts to remodel the bone so that they can restore stability. This may cause unwanted bony growths to build up, called osteophytes. The joint may become misshapen. This problem is often called osteoarthritis.

Osteoarthritis can also derive from previous harm to the joint like a fracture or previous irritation in the joint.

3. Soft tissue musculoskeletal pain

Smooth tissue musculoskeletal pain is felt in tissues apart from the important joints and bone fragments. The pain often impacts an integral part of the body pursuing damage or overuse, such as lateral epicondylitis, and hails from the muscles or smooth tissues assisting the joints.

Pain that is more widespread and associated with other symptoms may indicate fibromyalgia.

4. Back pain

Back again pain can arise from the muscles, discs, nerves, ligaments, bone fragments, or joints. Back again pain may stem from issues with organs inside your body. It may also be due to known pain, for example, whenever a problem somewhere else in the torso leads to pain in the trunk.

There could be a particular cause, such as osteoarthritis. This is called spondylosis when it occurs in the backbone. Imaging assessments or a physical exam may identify this.

A "slipped" disk is another reason behind back again pain, as is osteoporosis, or loss of the bone fragments.

If a health care provider cannot identify the precise reason behind back pain, it is referred to as "nonspecific" pain.

5. Connective tissue disease (CTD)

Connective tissues support, bind together, or individual other body tissues and organs. They include tendons, ligaments, and cartilage.

CTD involves joint pain and swelling. The inflammation could also take place in other cells, including the pores and skin, muscles, lungs, and kidneys. This may lead to various symptoms besides unpleasant joints, and it could require discussion with a variety of specialists.

Types of CTD include:

- SLE, or lupus

- scleroderma, or systemic sclerosis

- dermatomyositis.

6. Infectious arthritis

A bacterium, computer virus, or fungi that enters a joint will often cause inflammation.

Microorganisms that can infect joint parts include:

- Salmonella and Shigella, pass on through food poisoning or contamination

- chlamydia and gonorrhea, that are sexually transmitted diseases (STDs)

- hepatitis C, a blood-to-blood illness which may be pass on through shared fine needles or transfusions

- A joint infection can frequently be cleared with antibiotics or other antimicrobial medication. However, the joint disease will often become chronic, and joint harm may be irreversible if chlamydia has persisted for quite a while.

7. Metabolic arthritis

The crystals is a chemical substance created when your body reduces substances called purines. Purines are located in human cellular material and many foods.

Most the crystals dissolves in bloodstream and moves to the kidneys. Following that, it goes by out in urine. Some individuals have high degrees of uric, acidity because they either normally produce more than they want or their body cannot clear the crystals quickly enough.

Uric acid accumulates and accumulates in some individuals and forms needle-like crystals in the joint, leading to unexpected spikes of extreme joint pain or a gout attack.

Gout can either come and go ahead shows or become chronic if the crystals quantity aren't reduced.

It commonly impacts an individual joint or a little number of bones, like the big toe and hands. It usually impacts the extremities. One theory is that the crystals form in cooler bones, away from the primary warmth of your body.

A number of the more prevalent types of joint disease are discussed below.

8. Rheumatoid arthritis

Arthritis rheumatoid and osteoarthritis talk about some characteristics, however they will vary conditions.

Arthritis rheumatoid (RA) occurs when your body's

immune system episodes the tissue of your body, specifically connective tissues, resulting in joint inflammation, pain, and degeneration of the joint cells.

Cartilage is a flexible, connective tissues in joint parts that absorb the pressure and surprise created by motion like working and walking. In addition, it protects the bones and permits smooth movement.

Persistent irritation in the synovia leads to the degeneration of cartilage and bone. This may then business lead to joint deformity, pain, bloating, and redness.

RA can appear at any age group and it is associated with exhaustion and prolonged tightness after rest.

RA causes premature mortalityTrusted Source and impairment and it can bargain standard of living. Conditions it is associated with include cardiovascular diseases, such as ischemic cardiovascular disease and stroke.

Diagnosing RA early provides a better potential for learning how to control symptoms successfully. This may decrease the impact of the condition on standard of living.

9. Osteoarthritis

Osteoarthritis is a common degenerative osteo-arthritis that impacts the cartilageTrusted Source, joint coating and ligaments, and underlying bone of the joint.

The break down of these tissues eventually leads to pain and joint stiffness.

The joints frequently suffering from osteoarthritis are the ones that get heavy use, such as hips, knees, hands, the spine, the bottom of the thumb, and the best toe joint.

10. Childhood arthritis

This can make reference to lots of types of arthritis. Juvenile idiopathic joint disease (JIA), also called juvenile arthritis rheumatoid (JRA), is the most commonTrusted Source type.

Arthritis in child years can cause long term damage to joint parts, and there is absolutely no remedy. However, remission can be done, where time the condition remains inactive.

It might be thanks to disease fighting capability problems.

11. Septic arthritis

This is considered to affect between 2 and 10 people atlanta divorce attorneys 100,000 in the overall population. Among people who have RA, it could influence 30 to 70 people per 100,000.

Septic arthritis is a joint inflammation that results from a bacterial or fungal infection. It commonly impacts the leg and hip.

It could develop when bacterias or other disease-causing micro-organisms pass on through the bloodstream to a joint, or when the joint is directly infected with a microorganism through damage or surgery.

Bacterias such as Staphylococcus, Streptococcus, or Neisseria gonorrhoeae cause most instances of acute septic joint disease. Microorganisms such as Mycobacterium tuberculosis and Candidiasis cause chronic septic joint disease. That is less common than severe septic arthritis.

Septic arthritis might occur at any age. In babies, it may happen before the age group of three years. The hip is a common site of disease at this age group.

Septic arthritis is unusual from three years to adolescence. Children with septic joint disease are much more likely than adults to be contaminated with Group B Streptococcus or Haemophilus influenzae if indeed they never have been vaccinated.

The incidence of bacterial arthritis caused by infection with H. influenzae has reduced by around 70 percent to

80 percent because the use of the H. influenzae b (Hib) vaccine became common.

The next conditions boost the threat of developing septic arthritis:

- existing osteo-arthritis or damage.

- artificial joint implants.

- infection elsewhere in the torso.

- presence of bacterias in the blood.

- persistent illness or disease (such as diabetes, RA and sickle cell disease).

- intravenous (IV) or injection drug use.

- medications that suppress the disease fighting capability.

- recent joint injury.

- recent joint arthroscopy or other surgery.

- conditions such as HIV, that weaken immunity.

- Diabetes.

- older age

Septic arthritis is a rheumatologic emergency as it could lead to quick joint destruction. It could be fatal.

12. Fibromyalgia

Fibromyalgia affects around 4 millionTrusted Source adults in the U.S, or about 2 percent of the populace.

It usually begins during middle age group or after, but it make a difference children.

Fibromyalgia can involve:

- widespread pain.

- sleep disturbance.

- Fatigue.

- Depression.

- issues with thinking and remembering

The individual may experience abnormal pain processing, where they reacts strongly to something that other folks wouldn't normally find painful.

There can also be tingling or numbness in the hands and feet, pain in the jaw, and digestive problems.

The sources of fibromyalgia are unfamiliar, however, many factors have been loosely associated with disease onset:

- stressful or distressing events.
- post-traumatic stress disorder (PTSD).
- injuries thanks to repetitive movements.
- disease, for example viral infections.
- having lupus, RA, or chronic low energy syndrome.
- family history.
- obesity

It is more prevalent among females.

13. Psoriatic arthritis

Psoriatic arthritis is a joint problem that often occurs with a condition of the skin called psoriasis. It really is thought to have an effect on between 0.3 and 1 percent of the populace in the U.S., and between 6 and 42 percent of individuals with psoriasis.

Most people who've psoriatic joint disease and psoriasis develop psoriasis first and then psoriatic joint disease, but joint problems can on occasion occur before skin damage appear.

The exact reason behind psoriatic arthritis is as yet not known, but it seems to involve the disease fighting capability attacking healthy cells and tissue. The irregular immune system response causes swelling in the bones and an overproduction of epidermis cells. Harm to the joint parts can result.

Factors that raise the risk, include:

- having psoriasis
- family history
- being aged from 30 to 50 year

People who have psoriatic arthritis generally have a higher quantity of risk factorsTrusted Source for coronary disease than the overall population, including increased BMI, triglycerides, and C-reactive proteins.

14. Gout

Gout is a rheumatic disease that occurs when the crystals, or monosodium urate, form in body cells and liquids. It happens when your body produces too much the crystals or will not excrete enough the crystals.

Acute gout normally appears as a severely red, hot, and inflamed joint and severe pain.

Risk factors include:

- over weight or obesity.

- Hypertension.

- alcohol intake.

- use of diuretics.

- a diet abundant with meats and seafood.

- some typically common medicines.

- poor kidney function

Very long periods of remission are possible, accompanied by flares enduring from times to weeks. Sometimes it could be chronic. Recurrent episodes of severe gout can result in a degenerative form of chronic joint disease called gouty joint disease.

15. Sjögren's syndrome

Sjögren's syndrome can be an autoimmune disorder that sometimes occurs alongside RA and SLE. It requires the damage of glands that produce tears and saliva. This causes dryness in the mouth area and eye and in the areas that always need moisture, like the nose, neck, and skin.

Additionally, it may affect the bones, lungs, kidneys, arteries, digestive organs, and nerves.

Sjögren's symptoms typically impacts in adults aged 40 to 50 years, and especially women.

According to a report in Clinical and Experimental Rheumatology, in 40 to 50 percentTrusted Source of individuals with primary Sjögren's syndrome, the problem affects tissues apart from the glands.

It could impact the lungs, liver organ, or kidneys, or it might lead to pores and skin vasculitis, peripheral neuropathy, glomerulonephritis, and low degrees of a material known as C4. All of these indicate a connection between Sjögren's and the disease fighting capability.

If these cells are affected, there's a risky of developing

non-Hodgkin's lymphoma.

16. Scleroderma

Scleroderma identifies several diseases that affect connective tissues in the torso. The individual will have areas of hard, dried out epidermis. Some types make a difference the inner organs and small arteries.

Scar-like tissue accumulates in your skin and causes damage. The cause happens to be unidentified. It often impacts people between your age groups of 30 to 50 years, and it could take place with other autoimmune diseases, such as lupus.

Scleroderma impacts individuals differently. The problems include pores and skin problems, some weakness in the center, lung harm, gastrointestinal problems, and kidney failing.

17. Systemic lupus erythematosus (SLE)

SLE, often called lupus, can be an autoimmune disease where in fact the disease fighting capability produces antibodies to cellular material in the body leading toTrusted Source common inflammation and injury. The condition is seen as a periods of disease and remissions.

It could appear at any age group, but starting point is most likelyTrusted Source is between your age range of 15 and 45 years. For each and every one man who gets lupus, between 4 and 12 women can do so.

Lupus make a difference the joints, epidermis, brain, lungs, kidneys, arteries, and other tissue. Symptoms include exhaustion, pain or bloating in joints, pores and skin rashes, and fevers.

The reason remains unclear, but maybe it's associated with genetic, environmental, and hormonal factors.

Early signs

The symptoms of arthritis that appear and exactly how they appear vary widely, with respect to the type.

They are able to develop steadily or suddenly. As joint disease is frequently a chronic disease, symptoms will come and go, or persist as time passes.

However, anyone who encounters the following four key indicators should see a medical expert.

- Pain: Pain from joint disease can be constant, or it could come and go. It could affect only 1 part, or be experienced in many areas of the body.

- Swelling: In a few types of joint disease the skin on the affected joint becomes red and enlarged and seems warm to touch.

- Stiffness. Tightness is an average sign. With some types, this is most probably upon getting up each day, after seated at a table, or after seated in an automobile for a long period. With other styles, stiffness might occur after exercise, or it might be persistent..

- Difficulty moving a joint: If moving a joint or waking up from a seat is hard or painful, this may indicate joint disease or another joint problem.

Rheumatoid arthritis

RA is a systemic disease, so that it usually impacts the joint parts on both edges of your body equally. The bones of the wrists, fingertips, knees, ft and ankles will be the mostly affected.

Joint symptoms can include:

- morning stiffness, long lasting more than one hour

pain, often in the same joint parts on both edges of your body.

- loss of flexibility of bones, possibly with deformity

Other medical indications include:

- upper body pain when sucking in, thanks to pleurisy.
- dried out eyes and mouth, if Sjögren's syndrome

exists.

- eye burning up, itching, and discharge.

- nodules under your skin, usually an indicator of more serious disease.

- numbness, tingling, or burning up in the hands and feet.

- sleep difficulties

Osteoarthritis

Osteoarthritis is generally a consequence of deterioration on the joint parts. It will influence joints which have been overworked more than others. People who have osteoarthritis may go through the following symptoms:

- pain and rigidity in the joints.

- pain that becomes even worse after exercise or strain on the joint.

- massaging, grating, or crackling appear whenever a joint is moved.

- morning stiffness.

- pain that triggers sleep disturbances

Some individuals may have changes associated with osteoarthritis that arrive within an x-ray, however they do not experience the symptoms.

Osteoarthritis typically impacts some bones more than others, like the still left or right leg, make or wrist.

Childhood arthritis

Symptoms of years as a child arthritis include:

- a joint that is inflamed, red, or warm.

- a joint that is stiff or small in movement.

- limping or difficulty using an arm or leg.

- a sudden high fever that will come and go.

- a rash on the trunk and extremities that comes and complements the fever.

- symptoms throughout your body, such as pale epidermis, swollen lymph glands.

- generally appearing unwell

Juvenile RA can also cause vision problems including uveitis, iridocyclitis, or iritis. If attention symptoms do happen they range from:

- red eyes.

- eye pain, particularly when taking a look at light.

- vision changes.

Septic arthritis

Symptoms of septic joint disease occur rapidly.

There is certainly often:

- fever.

- intense joint pain that becomes more serious with movement.

- joint swelling in a single joint

Symptoms in newborns or newborns include:

- crying when the infected joint is moved.
- Fever.
- inability to go the limb with the infected joint.
- irritability

Symptoms in children and adults include:

- inability to go the limb with the infected joint.
- intense joint pain, inflammation, and redness

fever.

- Chills sometimes occur but are an uncommon indicator.

Fibromyalgia

Fibromyalgia may result in the followingTrusted Source symptoms:

- popular pain, often with specific soft points.

- sleep disturbance.

- Fatigue.

- psychological stress.

- morning stiffness.

- tingling or numbness in hands and feet.

- head aches, including migraines.

- irritable bowel syndrome.

- issues with thinking and memory space, sometimes called "fibro fog".

- Unpleasant menstrual periods and other pain syndromes

Psoriatic arthritis

Symptoms of psoriatic joint disease may be mild and involve just a few joint parts like the end of the fingertips or toes.

Severe psoriatic joint disease make a difference multiple

joints, like the backbone. Vertebral symptoms are usually sensed in the low backbone and sacrum. These contain stiffness, burning up, and pain.

People who have psoriatic arthritis frequently have your skin and toenail changes of psoriasis, and your skin gets even worse at exactly the same time as the joint disease.

Gout

Symptoms of gout involve:

- pain and inflammation, often in the best toe, leg, or ankle joint joints.

- unexpected pain, often at night time, which might be throbbing, crushing, or excruciating.

- warm and sensitive important joints that appear red and swollen.

- fever sometimes occurs

After having gout for quite some time, an individual can

develop tophi. Tophi are lumps below your skin, typically round the bones or obvious on fingertips and ear. Multiple, small tophi may develop, or a big white lump. This may cause deformation and extending of your skin.

Sometimes, tophi burst and drain spontaneously, oozing a white, chalky material. Tophi that are starting to break through your skin can result in infections or osteomyelitis. Some patients will require immediate surgery to drain the tophus.

Sjögren's syndrome

Symptoms of Sjögren's symptoms include:

- dried out and itchy eye, and a sense that something is in the attention.

- dry mouth.

- difficulty swallowing or eating.

- lack of sense of taste.

- problems speaking.

- solid or stringy saliva.

- mouth area sores or pain.

- Hoarseness.

- Fatigue.

- Fever.

- change in color of hands or feet.

- joint pain or joint swelling.

- swollen glands

Scleroderma

Symptoms of scleroderma can include:

- fingers or feet that change blue or white in response to winter, known as Raynaud's phenomenon.

- hair loss.

- pores and skin that becomes darker or lighter than normal.

- tightness and tightness of epidermis on the fingertips, hands, forearm, and face.

- small white lumps under the skin that sometimes ooze a white substance that appears like toothpaste.

- sores or ulcers on the fingertips or toes.

- limited and mask-like pores and skin on the facial skin.

- numbness and pain in your toes.

- pain, rigidity, and inflammation of the wrist, fingertips, and other joints.

- dried out cough, shortness of breath, and wheezing.

- gastrointestinal problems, such as bloating after meals, constipation, and diarrhea.

- difficulty swallowing.

- esophageal reflux or heartburn

Systemic lupus erythematosus (SLE)

The most frequent signs of SLE, or lupus, are:

- red rash or color change on the facial skin, often in the form of the butterfly over the nose and cheeks.

- painful or enlarged joints.

- unexplained fever.

- upper body pain when deep breathing deeply.

- swollen glands.

- extreme fatigue.

- unusual hair loss.

- pale or crimson fingers or feet from chilly or stress.

- sensitivity to sunlight.

- low bloodstream count.

- depressive disorder, trouble thinking or storage problems.

Chapter 3

9 Herbs to Battle Arthritis Pain

1. Aloe vera

Aloe vera is one of the very most commonly used herbal products in option medicine. Known because of its curing properties, it's popular for dealing with small epidermis abrasions. You might curently have a container of aloe vera gel in the medication cupboard from a previous sunburn. This same kind of product may be employed topically to soothe aching joint parts.

Aloe vera is also available entirely form from the leaves of the vegetable. The National Middle for Complementary and Integrative Health (NCCIH)Trusted Source says that dental aloe vera can cause reduced blood glucose and gastrointestinal aspect results, such as diarrhea. Topical aloe vera, on the other hands, will not cause any part effects and really should be safe to try for joint disease. Purchase topical aloe vera now.

2. Boswellia

Boswellia, also known as frankincense, is praised by alternate medicine practitioners because of its anti-inflammatory features. It's produced from the gum of boswellia trees and shrubs indigenous to India.

This herb is considered to work by blocking substances (leukotrienes) that attack healthy joints in autoimmune diseases such as RA. The NCCIHTrusted Source acknowledges encouraging proof boswellia in pet studies. Nonetheless it notes too little human tests. Boswellia comes in tablet form and skin medications.

3. Cat's claw

Cat's claw is another anti-inflammatory herb that may reduce swelling in joint disease. This plant is from a tropical vine, and its own usage goes back to Incan civilizations. Typically, cat's claw is utilized to improve the disease fighting capability.

Lately, the immunity powers of the herb have been tried in arthritis. The downside is that cat's claw may overstimulate the disease fighting capability and make joint disease pain worse.

Based on the Arthritis Foundation, a report demonstrated cat's claw can help with RA bloating. But there's no evidence that this plant can prevent further joint harm.

4. Eucalyptus

Like aloe vera, eucalyptus is accessible in Western marketplaces. It's found in oral medicaments, and topical essential oil components are used for a number of conditions. Topical types of eucalyptus leaves are accustomed to treat joint disease pain.

The plant leaves contain tannins, which might be helpful in reducing swelling and the pain arthritis causes. Some users follow-up with warmth pads to increase the consequences of eucalyptus on inflamed joints.

Make sure to test yourself for allergies before using topical eucalyptus. Put a little amount of the merchandise on your forearm. When there is no response in 24 to 48 hours, it ought to be safe to use.

5. Ginger

You might have ginger in your spice cabinet for cooking food, but this herb is also a staple in a variety of medicine cabinets. The same substances that provide ginger its strong taste likewise have anti-inflammatory properties.

The NCCIH says that early studies in reducing joint swelling with ginger in RA are promising. But more human being trials are had a need to better understand its action. In folk medication and Chinese medication ginger can be used to increase blood flow, which brings temperature and curing properties to the affected area. Research shows guarantee for the utilization of ginger in every types of joint disease.

6. Green tea

Green tea extract is one of the very most popular drinks in the world, and has been used to lessen inflammation in the torso. It's possible that green tea extract may be used to treat joint disease inflammation by means of drinks, tablets, or tinctures.

Inside a 2010 research, the NCCIH discovered that green tea will help people who have osteoarthritis (OA) and RA. But a lot more studies remain needed to show the potential advantages of green tea.

7. Thunder god vine

Thunder god vine is one of the oldest herbs found in Chinese medication. Components from skinned origins are recognized for suppressing an overactive disease fighting capability. This makes thunder god vine a possible alternate treatment for autoimmune diseases such as RA. It's better to apply right to your skin in a topical form. Thunder god vine may work best along with standard RA medications.

Use extreme care with this natural herb, as possible poisonous if extracts derive from the areas of the vine. Long-term useTrusted Source is not suggested.

8. Turmeric

Turmeric is a yellowish powder created from the related flowering seed. It's found in food preparation to make curry. In addition, it has anti-inflammatory properties.

Laboratory studies on rats also have found this vitamin may gradual the development of RA. Curcumin, the active component in turmeric, has been found in folk medication for a long time. Unlike other styles of herbal remedies, the NCCIH found turmeric may work best in fighting joint pain when used orally.

There still must be more tests done on the safety of

turmeric, but its use is promising.

9. Willow bark

Using willow bark is one of the oldest treatments for inflammation. Actually, people during Hippocrates' time (5th hundred years B.C.) chewed on willow bark to help treat inflammatory conditions.

One research reported that the plant shows guarantee in relieving OA-related joint pain, particularly in the legs, back, sides, and throat. This treatment is used orally, either by tea or tablet.

Obtaining the right dose is vital. An overdose can cause rashes and other kinds of inflammation. Usually do not use willow bark invest the bloodstream thinners or are allergic to aspirin.

Ask your physician about complementary medicine

Given the increased prevalence of herbal medicine, conventional general practitioners are more willing to evaluate the advantages of alternative remedies. When dealing with arthritis, a few of these natural herbs may complement your present medications. But it's important to comprehend that herbal products can cause serious aspect effects.

It's also important to learn that herbs aren't monitored for quality, purity, product packaging, or dose by the FDA. You'll be able to have polluted products or inactive elements, so buy herbal remedies from an established source.

Discuss all joint disease treatment plans with your physician and don't stop taking recommended medications unless instructed. Also, retain in brain that complementary medication isn't exclusive to herbs. Other complementary methods to arthritis treatment include:

- massages.

- ice or high temperature packs.

- aerobic exercise.

- tai chi.

- Yoga.

- shower and soaking therapies.

- stress management like biofeedback and meditation.

- a healthy diet plan which include omega-3 essential fatty acids.

- vitamin D vitamins if your vitamin D quantity are low.

- Acupuncture.

- supportive shoes.

- weight management

Acknowledgements

The Glory of this book success goes to God Almighty and my beautiful Family, Fans, Readers & well-wishers, Customers, and Friends for their endless support and encouragement.

www.ingramcontent.com/pod-product-compliance
Lightning Source LLC
Chambersburg PA
CBHW020303030426
42336CB00010B/887